Survival Medicine:

Handbook That Will Save Your Life Before Ambulance Come!

Table Of Content

Introduction

I would like to thank and congratulate you on downloading *"Survival Medicine: Handbook that Will Save Your Life Before Ambulance Come!"* This book is a great handbook that offers you all kinds of tips and suggestions on how you can prepare survival medicine in an emergency. Gaining this knowledge and skills will certainly be most beneficial if you find yourself in a wilderness where you have perhaps lost contact with civilization and must rely on your own first aid skills to survive this ordeal you may find yourself in.

You just never know when you could find yourself in a situation where you need to do some basic first aid on yourself or others while waiting for an ambulance to arrive or medical help of some sort. It is very important when you are going outside of the protection of civilization to explore the wilderness. During times like this it is vital that you and your group have prepared by making sure to bring a first aid kit on your adventure. I am sure you will find the tips and suggestions within these pages most helpful to you in helping to guide you on how to prepare emergency survival medicine and treatments.

Chapter 1. Building Your Basic First Aid Kit

If you find yourself in a medical emergency when in the wilderness, it is vital that you are prepared to help ensure that you will have the best tolls available. You can build your own first aid kit or you can purchase a prepared kit. You should make sure that your first aid kit has the following items included in it:

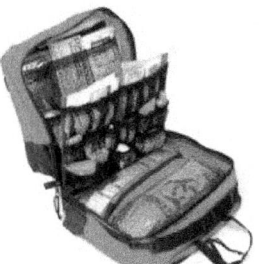

- Latex gloves, have lots of pairs as you do not want to re-use them.
- Roll of 1-inch wide athletic tape. Bring about 1 roll per person. It works great for dressing wounds, prevents blisters, and will help to support joints such as twisted ankle.
- Rolled gauze to maintain a dressing for wounds.
- Sterile wrapped gauze pads in variety of sizes. Make sure to have some that are non-adherent, as they are suitable for certain types of wounds.
- Scissors
- Tweezers
- A tourniquet
- Over the counter meds such as topical antibiotic cream, gastrointestinal medications, anti-diarrheal, pain relievers, antihistamines, and stomach soothing medications. Pack your kit in a waterproof container.

Wound Care
When faced with a wound in the wilderness, there are two initial priorities: controlling the bleeding, and preventing infection. Bleeding must be controlled quickly to help minimize the chance of the injured person going into shock or dying from blood loss.

Infection must be prevented from setting into the wound, so that bacteria will not multiply and make the injured party sick.

Control Bleeding

If there is a wound that is bleeding freely take a gauze and apply pressure to the wound with it. If possible try to elevate the wound above the height of the individual's heart, this will help to slow the blood flow. If the pressure is not stopping the bleeding, you may need to apply a tourniquet. Using a tourniquet should only be used as a last resort. The use of tourniquets can result in the need for an amputation or other complications. However, if the risk of death due to blood loss is a threat, and other methods are not working a tourniquet is necessary.

Infection Prevention

Once you have managed to control the bleeding, it is very important to take proactive steps to make sure that infection is prevented. These steps include cleaning the wound with soap and water, rinsing it clear of any foreign objects, using tweezers if needed. Keep irrigating the wound with water, and rinsing it with iodine.

Treating Shock

A person will go into medical shock due to loss of blood or insufficient blood flow throughout their body as well as other severe physiological stress. Blood loss, trauma, dehydration, head injury, and severe infections are just a few of the many situations which lead to a person going into shock.

Diagnosing Shock

You can tell if a person has gone into shock based on the following typical symptoms:

- Skin is pale

- Dizziness, disorientation, agitation
- Excessive thirst
- Hyperventilation
- Fainting

Treatment

If you believe that someone is going into shock, it is vital that you treat them. Shock can be life threatening if not treated. Below are some basic steps for treatment of shock:

1. Place the person suffering from shock onto their back. Elevate their legs six to eight inches above the level of their heart. If the person is unconscious, make sure to place them on their side or lying on their stomach with their head turned to the side. This is to help ensure that they will not choke on vomit or other fluids.

2. Any wet clothing the person is wearing remove it, and ensure they are comfortable. If it is cold weather, use blankets and other heat sources to warm the injured person. If it is hot out, try and find a shady spot for the person.

3. If the person is conscious keep them hydrated by giving them fluids, preferably containing salt or sugar.

4. Allow the person to get some rest until they recover.

When to Evacuate

If you do experience injury or illness while in the wilderness, it is a good idea to add an evacuation plan or have one in place. Make sure that you tell friends and family where you are going to be or location. This is important because you may not be able to contact them in an emergency so they need to know where to begin searching for you. If you do get contact, ask what is the best way for you to approach medical treatment.

Chapter 2. First Aid Vs. Survival Medicine

There is a difference between caring for an injured person after an earthquake, until the first responders arrive to caring for that person from the start of them becoming injured or sick right through until they make their recovery. There are many first aid courses offered for the public to take. In the US, most volunteer ambulance departments are constantly looking for new recruits. The Red Cross teaches first aid, in many countries, often with a focus on disasters.

If you want to give your first aid knowledge a good boost, seeking out such a course would be a great idea.

First Aid

First aid is the immediate response to an emergency or sudden illness. It helps to save the patient, ensuring that they will be given the best treatment to help ensure that they will survive the ordeal they are in.

First aid is a very essential skill, it is your immediate response to a serious medical problem. You will need to diagnose the problem, and remove any immediate dangers that could cause further damage or even death to the victim.

If you find yourself in the middle of an emergency, you will follow the strategy known to first responders: stabilize the patient and ready them for transportation. You will prepare the victim to be transported to a medical facility where they will be able to get more in depth treatment.

Outback Medicine

Not all disasters happen within a civilized region. You could be involved in a plane crash, where you are asked to help provide aid for other passengers. If you are stranded somewhere far from civilization, you might become the only hope that the injured person has for surviving. You will need to factor in the follow-up care to keep the injured party stable until help does arrive.

Survival Medicine

The third scenario is where it is assumed that help is not coming. This would be a safe assumption in a situation where you are in the middle of a large-scale disaster that has cut you off from civilization or you are one of very few survivors. In this scenario, you are needed at the site of the initial injury. Not only are you going to have to stabilize the injury, but you will need to continue your care until the injured party is cured or controlled.

You will need to know how to tackle chronic conditions such as thyroid and arthritis problems, heart disease and chicken pox. Survival medicine is an all-encompassing skill with a different approach to basic first aid.

First Aid Strategy

When you are a first responder to an accident, illness, or injury, there is a basic order of duties that you must follow. As the first responder, you are the primary caregiver, whether it is a full collapse of civilization or a car crash, it is your job to see that you and your patient emerge in the best condition possible given the circumstances that you are in.

It is important that you and your patient's safety is important, so the set of principles that you follow will be your mantra. When you find, yourself faced with a need to employ your first aid skills, whether it is until help arrives or for the long term, the following are steps you must follow:

1. Assess the situation. Study the scene you are faced with, be on the look-out for any dangers or hazards that could put you or your patient at risk. For example, make sure that you will not be hit by falling debris while you are trying to reach your patient.

2. Remove immediate dangers. To help ensure that the situation does not become even worse, make sure to remove any immediate dangers before you begin to administer treatment. Remember that your own safety is just as important as your patient's safety. If you too, become injured their chances of survival are greatly reduced or lost all together. Put out fires, and remove debris, move your patient to a safer location if you cannot secure the scene itself.

3. Protect yourself from becoming contaminated. Since you do not know fully what you are dealing with, protect yourself before you administer aid. Using a mask, gloves and apron are very important medical tools, not only will they help to prevent contaminated fluids from contacting you, but they will also protect your patient from becoming contaminated from your body.

4. Assess for life threatening injuries. What you need to assess right away if there is anything that could be threatening your patient's life. There is no use spending time diagnosing a compound fracture, for example, if your patient in the meantime is bleeding out due to a severed artery. You will need to check the following:

Airway—is there anything that could be preventing your patient from inhaling oxygen? Check to make sure that there are no objects in their mouth or throat that are blocking their airway.

Breathing—check to make sure that your patient is breathing normally.

Circulation—is your patient breathing normally? Check to see if there is any severe bleeding that could be life threatening to your patient.

Extreme injury—check to see if your patient has a neck or head injury that needs to be stabilized to help ensure their survival.

Exposure—is your patient exposed to an environmental or any external threat that could be life threatening?

5. Treat life threatening issues. You must immediately deal with any life-threatening issues, before you continue with your diagnosis and first aid. Before you begin a deeper examination of your patient, it is vital that you get them stabilized first.

6. Perform a thorough examination of situation. The injured person may not be able to communicate to you their injuries, because they might be unconscious. If they are conscious ask them what happened, and where they are hurt. This will offer you some help in diagnosing the situation, but keep in mind that your patient may not be aware of all their injuries. Some injuries can cause paralysis or numbness. When you examine the patient's body more thoroughly it will help you to become aware of the less obvious injuries.

7. Administer aid. Perform first aid on your patient's injuries, as well as treating them for things such as shock and hypothermia. Your goal here is to stabilize the patient and give them the best chance for recovery. Except in extreme conditions, the patient's long term care will take place in another location.

8. Make plans to evacuate. If help is on the way you will not have to worry about transporting your patient. However, if you need to transport them to a safe location, you need to plan to do this in such a way to prevent any part of the patient's injuries worsening in the process.

9. Transport the patient. First you need to make sure that your patient is stable and secure before you attempt to move them. This is especially true when you are dealing with a neck or back injury, moving the person could cause severe damage. You might have to create a shelter where you are so that you can treat the patient in place. If you feel that the patient is stable enough to move, make sure that any broken limbs are secured, and bandages will stay in place.

Chapter 3. The Principles of First Response

While you are following, the guidelines covered in the previous chapter to successfully treat your patient at the scene of the accident or their injury, you need to follow a set of principles. These principles will help you to improve your chances of success—and can leave your patient in the best condition possible. Here is a guideline of principles to try and follow: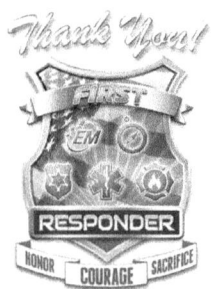

- **Remain calm.** It is not always easy to remain calm, but it is imperative. By remaining calm you will make better decisions, and will be aware of more details and will certainly be more productive when you are in a calm state of mind. When we hurry and rush through things we often make more mistakes. We also must keep in mind what your reaction will have on the patient. The last thing you want to do is cause the patient to become even more panicked than they are ready are. It could cause them to move and in the process, could add to their injuries and also have a negative effect on their heart rate.

- **Involve the patient.** Keeping your patient involved is important, because they are more aware of what happened to them than you are. Their help can be invaluable when it comes to you treating their injuries. The patient can also inform you of hidden issues, for example, a blood clotting disease that could increase the time it will take for the wound to heal. They can inform you if they have a headache or they feel nauseated, you cannot see these, but they can help you in your diagnosis. When you involve the patient, it can help to keep them calm and quell their fears. It is a show of respect to ask the patient's permission before you begin treatment and to explain your progress as you go. Keep in mind that it is not your body and you have no right to touch it. It is best, if possible to seek the permission to do so from the patient first.

- **Seek information.** Even if your patient is unable to communicate with you, there are still clues you can search for. Assess the scene, try to figure out what led to these injuries, and why?

  It can often help you to give a better diagnosis or even allow you to spot more subtle injuries to the patient. Check the patient for medical cards or bracelets that may alert you to pre-existing medical conditions.

- **Assume the worst.** Pessimism in a first aid situation is certainly useful. It is a good idea to assume that the patient has serious injuries such as a broken neck or back. Better that you go the extra mile to move a patient onto a stretcher than to discover too late, as you help them to stand, that a neck injury was present all along.

- **Enlist help.** Speed can certainly be an important criterion, especially if you are in a crisis, and you need to get the patient to a safe location as quickly as possible. Other people may not be medically trained, but they still can assist you with many of the tasks you may need to perform. It is seldom a good idea to move a patient on your own, unless you have no choice.

- **Take charge.** If you are enlisting help, make sure that you establish yourself as being the medical authority in the situation. Explain to others that you are taking charge of the situation, as a first responder and have the situation under control. Use an authoritative tone, and request assistance from others, explaining what you need and why. You can relinquish your authority if you discover that there are more qualified medical professionals within the group. It is never a bad idea to defer to greater knowledge and experience.

- **Consider all dangers.** Accidents rarely happen in safe areas. Falls, crashes, and even disasters—these things have potential to harm you or anyone else on the scene. Never put yourself in harm's way or anyone else without good reason. For example, throwing yourself into a river filled with rapids is not going to save the victim. Always be on the alert for dangers, while treating the patient, move everyone to a safe location.

- **Think hard before moving the patient.** Before you consider moving from the scene, make sure that the patient is recovered enough to be moved. Injuries could become more serious if a patient is moved. One of the most difficult choices you may have to make is deciding whether to move your patient. You need to gather as much information as you can before you even consider moving them.

Chapter 4. First Aid & Medical Supplies

If you are the person that is responsible for first aid within your group, you will be responsible for making sure that your kit bag is equipped to administer care. You need to have enough supplies to last for the time where you will be unable to receive help from a medical facility.

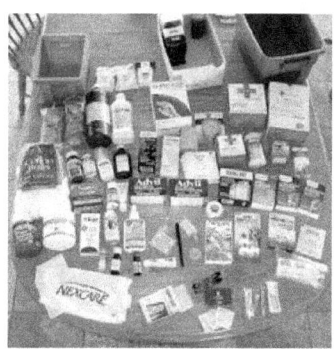

If you are heading out on an excursion with a group, you need to make sure that you have enough medical supplies to last a few days, before help can arrive. If you are stocking a shelter that you are planning to use as a residence after a disaster or collapse, you will need to stock it up with months, if not years of supplies.

For those everyday maladies and small aches and pains, you will need:

- Aspirin for aches and pains and heart problems
- Painkillers (also have a child friendly version if you have young children)
- Benadryl for allergic reactions
- Flu and severe cold remedies
- Diarrhea medicine
- Adrenaline injectors
- Antibiotics
- Women's feminine hygiene products
- Diapers for baby and other care products for infants
- Stomach upset remedy

- Good quality skin lotion
- Calamine lotion
- Burn gel or spray
- Aloe Vera gel for sunburn
- Potassium iodide tablets
- Silver sulfadiazine cream
- Soap and hand sanitizer
- Celox combat gauze
- Topical antifungal powder or ointment
- Steroid cream
- Antihistamines
- A supply of any medications that you or others in your family or party, take regularly such as insulin or heart medication.

For treatment of wounds and other emergencies:

- Plenty of bandages, they will need to be changed regularly
- Band Aids and dressings
- Hemostatic products for serious bleeds
- A hemostat clamp
- Scalpels and a field knife
- Splints and wraps for all limbs in case of breakages and sprains
- Towels
- Disinfectant, such as rubbing alcohol to clean wounds
- Medical tape
- Medical grade glue
- Eye pads
- A neck clamp
- A neck collar
- An epinephrine auto injector for severe allergic reaction

- Anticoagulant
- Activated charcoal
- Asthma inhaler
- A nylon suture
- Corticosteroid tablets

General equipment for your medical room:

- A small flashlight
- Scissors
- Tweezers
- Sterilizing wipes for cleaning wounds
- A tourniquet
- Syringes and injection needles
- Scalpels and scalpel blades of various sizes
- A surgical mask for use during first aid and surgery
- A stethoscope
- A thermometer—one oral and one rectal
- Pen light or head lamp
- A stretcher
- Crutches
- Cold and hot compresses for swelling
- A thermal blanket for treating hypothermia
- Compression wraps
- A blood pressure cuff
- A glucose meter
- Cotton balls
- Petroleum jelly
- Safety pins
- Medical needle and thread for stitching wounds

Many of these items you can purchase in pharmacies and supermarkets or online. After a disaster locate the nearest medical supply center near your location. It is never recommended to administer such treatments under normal circumstances without having proper medical training, but when in a disaster scenario this calls for different behavior.

Chapter 5. Checking for Immediate Signals & Vital Signs

When you first encounter a patient, do not assume that you are seeing the full extent of their injuries. The patient may not complain of nothing more than a sprained ankle, but that does not mean you are safe to assume that there is nothing else wrong with the patient. We have all heard of internal bleeding stories, that have gone unnoticed until it was too late or the broken ankle that was walked on for two days before anyone realized it was more than just a sprained ankle.

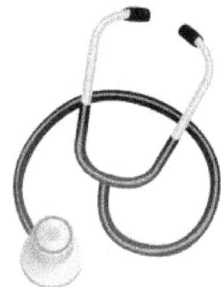

As a first responder, you need to assess the patient's full body, from head to toe. You need to assume the worst—an injury is guilty until it the first responder has proven it innocent. Checking your patient's vital signs is going to be your primary indicator of your patient's status. Checking to see if your patient's breathing, heart beat and blood pressure are all good. When you are starting your assessment of your patient these are the details you are going to want to stay focused on.

The vital signs of your patient will vary according to their age. In general, look for vital signs within the following ranges:

- Expect 30 to 50 breaths per minute from a newborn baby, a pulse between 120 to 160 beats per minute and blood pressure of 60 to 80.
- Expect 30 to 40 breaths per minute from a baby aged six months to a year, a pulse between 110 to 140 beats per minute, and blood pressure of 70 to 80.
- Expect 20 to 30 breaths from a toddler aged two to four, a pulse between 100 and 110 beats per minute, and blood pressure of 80 to 95.

- Expect 14 to 20 breaths per minute from a child between five and eight years old, a pulse between 90 and 100 beats per minute, and blood pressure of 90 to 100.
- Expect 12 to 20 breaths per minute from a child between the ages of eight and twelve years old, a pulse between 80 and 100 per minute, and blood pressure of 100 to 110.
- Expect 12 to 20 breaths per minute from a teenager between the ages of 12 to 18, with a pulse between 60 to 90 beats per minute, and blood pressure of 100 to 120.
- Expect 12 to 18 breaths per minute from an adult, with a pulse between 55 to 90 beats per minute, and blood pressure of 120.

You need to check off all the likely indicators of a problem when you first examine your patient. As a general rule try to follow these steps while you investigate the status of your patient's health:

1. Check for breathing: If your patient is unconscious, place your ear near to the nose and mouth to see if you can hear breath coming in and out. Watch their chest at the same time. Count the breaths according to your patient's vital signs. If the patient is not breathing or is struggling for breath, you will need to open the airway or breathe on their behalf. It is vital to steady the breathing as your patient will not be able to go without oxygen. If you hear strange sounds, such as rattling, there could be an obstruction in the throat that you will need to remove.

2. Check your patient's pulse. Using the tip of your middle finger and index fingers check for a pulse on the artery at the patient's wrist. If you are unable to locate one, check the inside of the upper arm (brachial artery), groin (femoral artery), or neck (carotid artery). If you cannot locate a pulse you will need to begin chest compressions immediately.

3. Look for bleeding. You should always check the heartbeat and breathing first with an unconscious patient. A conscious patient clearly has these functions to at least be good enough to be capable of speech. When you are dealing with a conscious patient, it is vital that you begin a dialogue with them immediately to help reassure them that they will be taken care of, and assure them of your intentions. Keep and eye out for any bleeding. Any sign of bleeding can be harmful, but it can be deadly if it is uncontrolled heavy bleeding. Examine the body of your patient to identify any areas that might be bleeding. These areas must be addressed as soon as possible.

4. Perform a full body evaluation of your patient. Move clothing around as much as you can without exposing the patient. Check for abnormalities on your patient's body, these could indicate fractures, wounds or other issues.

5. Check your patient's mental status. If your patient is awake, ask them questions to find out how lucid they are, such as their name, profession, and date. Listen to your patient's speech: if there is an abnormality such as slurring, this could be a symptom of a problem such as hypothermia.

6. Check your patient's blood pressure. When a person is at rest their average blood pressure should be 140/190. If it is too low this could indicate that your patient is in shock or is hemorrhaging.

7. Feel your patient's neck. Carefully and gently check your patient's vertebra and look for tenderness and muscles in spasm. Check their Adam's apple for a sensation almost like crunching. If you suspect that your patient has suffered a neck injury, immobilize the neck as quickly as possible. Sudden movements could exacerbate the problem and pain could cause your patient to twitch or try to move.

8. Check your patient's spine. Run your fingers down your patient's spine to check for back injuries. Press gently as you go down the spine, checking for tender areas. Ask your patient to move their limbs, and ask them if they have lost feeling in any areas. You can lightly pinch fingers and toes to see if your patient still has sensation. If there is loss of feeling this could indicate a back injury. This will require your patient to be immobilized as securely as possible—and kept in one position.

9. Check your patient for head injuries. Check the skull by pressing lightly around it to look for any areas on the skull or skin that are raised or depressed or are bleeding. Shine a light into your patient's eyes to make sure that both pupils are the same size and are responding to the light by constricting. If the pupils are small in your patient this could be a sign of an overdose or a brain injury. Pupils that are uneven can mean that the eye itself is injured or that your patient has a head injury. Check for other injuries on the head such as broken teeth, nose or swollen tongue.

10. Examine your patient's skin. Check for indicators such as abnormal skin color, bruises, bites, rashes or burns. Feel the temperature of your patient to check for fever. Press down on fingernails to check for circulation, pressing down will cause the skin to go white; if the circulation is normal, color will return to skin in two seconds.

If you pinch the skin and it remains loose, this could be an indication that your patient is dehydrated. Check inside of your patient's eyelids for a pale color that can indicate that there is internal bleeding or anemia.

11. Check your patient's chest. Check the chest area for any deformities, also observe the expanding and contracting of each breath that your patient takes.

12. Examine your patient's abdomen. Check for cuts and wounds, also press to see if there is any tenderness.

13. Check your patient's limbs and joints. Check each limb by pressing to check for tenderness, as well as the chest, ribs and collarbone.

14. Check your patient's temperature. By checking your patient's temperature this can indicate to you that not all is well with the patient's body. If your patient's temperature is too low this could indicate that they are suffering from hypothermia, while too high could mean hyperthermia or fever.

Whether you need to keep your patient from moving or not, it is best to assume that the situation will deteriorate with time. Repeat your examinations regularly, looking for new signs and signals, check to see if the symptoms that you are treating are not worsening or spreading.

Keep checking the mental status of your patient to make sure that they remain lucid. Do not leave your patient alone, if you need to get more supplies, ask someone to sit with your patient while you are gone.

Taking a first aid course is something that you will certainly not regret, as you will be taught how to treat injured people for many kinds of injuries, wounds, and other medical conditions. You will be instructed by medical professionals on how to perform such first aid treatments as CPR, Mouth to Mouth Resuscitation, Treat Shock, Recovery Position and much more first aid skills. These are certainly great skills to have especially when we live in such a world of uncertainty, we just don't know when and where the next disaster will strike. It will certainly feel good to know that you have prepared yourself for the worst, it is better to be safe than sorry. Learning these first responder skills will make you feel more secure knowing that you will be able to help those in need during an emergency.

Conclusion

I hope that you will find the tips and suggestions, on how to prepare for becoming a good first responder in an emergency useful to you in your time of need. I am sure that you will be happy that you learned these first aid skills and made the effort to be prepared for an emergency. You will gain much comfort in knowing that you are armed with the proper medical supplies and knowledge to be able to help others in need of your assistance in an emergency. A good start for preparing yourself would be to start by putting together your own emergency first aid kit.

I would like to thank you once again for downloading my book, your support of my work means a great deal to me. I would love to read a review of my book by you on Amazon. Take care and a I wish you great success in you developing your first responder skills.

FREE BonusReminder

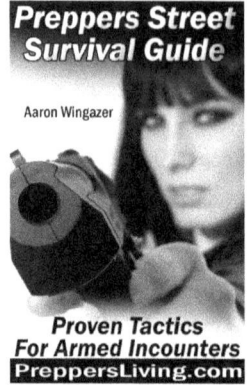

If you have not grabbed it yet, please go ahead and download your special bonus report
"Preppers Street Survival Guide: Proven Tactics For Armed Incounters"

SimplyClicktheButtonBelow

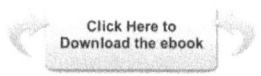

OR **Go to This Page**

http://preppersliving.com/free

BONUS #2: More Free & Discounted Books & Products

Do you want to receive more Free/Discounted Books or Products?

We have a mailing list where we send out our new Books or Products when
they go free or with a discount on Amazon. Click on the link below to sign up
for Free & Discount Book & Product Promotions.

=> Sign Up for Free & Discount Book & Product Promotions <=

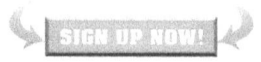

OR Go to this URL

http://zbit.ly/1WBb1Ek

www.ingramcontent.com/pod-product-compliance
Lightning Source LLC
Chambersburg PA
CBHW072013280526
45788CB00005B/2022